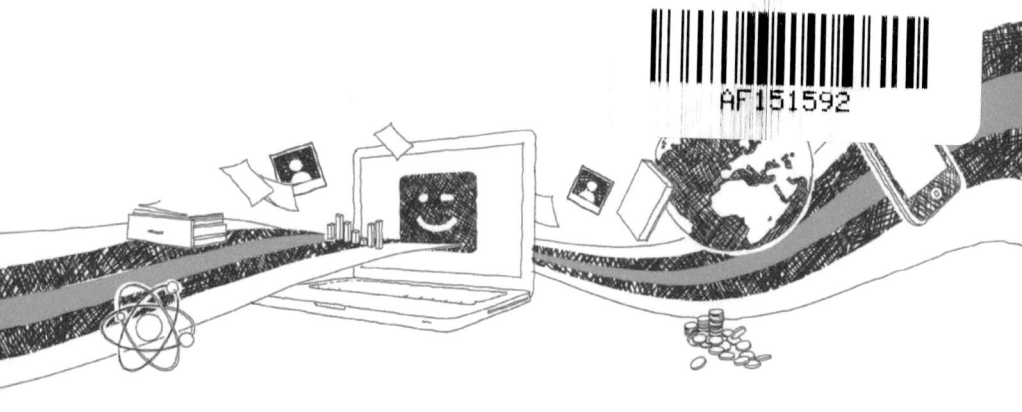
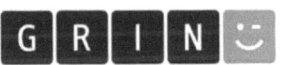

Petra Heyen

Regulatory Intelligence as the Basis for Regulatory Strategy and Global Drug Development

GRIN Publishing

Bibliographic information published by the German National Library:

The German National Library lists this publication in the National Bibliography; detailed bibliographic data are available on the Internet at http://dnb.dnb.de .

Imprint:

Copyright © 2004 GRIN Verlag GmbH
Print and binding: Books on Demand GmbH, Norderstedt Germany
ISBN: 978-3-640-86257-3

This book at GRIN:

http://www.grin.com/en/e-book/38005/regulatory-intelligence-as-the-basis-for-regulatory-strategy-and-global

GRIN - Your knowledge has value

Since its foundation in 1998, GRIN has specialized in publishing academic texts by students, college teachers and other academics as e-book and printed book. The website www.grin.com is an ideal platform for presenting term papers, final papers, scientific essays, dissertations and specialist books.

Visit us on the internet:

http://www.grin.com/

http://www.facebook.com/grincom

http://www.twitter.com/grin_com

Regulatory Intelligence as the Basis for Regulatory Strategy and Global Drug Development

Wissenschaftliche Prüfungsarbeit

zur Erlangung des Titels

„Master of Drug Regulatory Affairs"

der Mathematisch-Naturwissenschaftlichen Fakultät

der Rheinischen Friedrich-Wilhelms-Universität Bonn

vorgelegt von

Dr. Petra Heyen

aus Vechta

Bonn 2004

Regulatory Intelligence as the basis for Regulatory Strategy and Global Drug Development

Dr. Petra Heyen (2004)

Language: English

Summary

The Regulatory Affairs department is a key discipline in the global network of drug development. During drug development, regulatory strategy is one crucial success factor for the approval of the development candidate. Also, regulatory strategy can optimise labelling in the key countries in order to maximise the market success. No submission and approval would be possible without the appropriate dossier composition and compilation. Without adherence to the respective guidance documents and scientific advice from Health Authorities to design the optimal clinical development plan, optimal labelling would not be feasible. These two examples show some characteristics of the regulatory strategy: it is highly interactive with other disciplines (e.g. clinical development plan based on the scientific advice from a Health Authority which has been arranged according to the regulatory rules) and it is heavily based on a thorough intelligence work (e.g. knowledge of relevant guidance documents, regulatory environment, competitor analysis) which enables the Regulatory Affairs Manager to know the "rules of the game" and to develop the optimal regulatory strategy for the current development candidate. The major cornerstone for developing a regulatory strategy is regulatory intelligence.

This document focuses on regulatory intelligence. The regulatory contributions to the global drug development from early research to submission are described. Strategies for generic drugs as well as detailed strategies for life-cycle management are excluded.

Major components of regulatory intelligence are:
* Competitor Information
* Information on Regulatory Environment
* Information on Legal Requirements

Competitor analysis is an essential aspect of the intelligence work. Sources of competitive information as well as relevant items of competitive information are described.

Sources of information about the regulatory environment (e.g. agency benchmarks, regulatory guidance documents and changes, trade associations, regulatory associations, ICH and WHO) and sources of information about the legal regulatory environment (general requirements, specific populations, orphan drug designation) are described and their tremendous impact on setting up and modifying the regulatory strategy evaluated.

Special attention is paid to the components and sources of regulatory intelligence information (e.g. Internet links and documents related to intelligence information). Some examples show how regulatory intelligence information supports the regulatory strategic considerations.

The last section describes the regulatory strategy itself and examples of how regulatory intelligence acts as the basis for setting up the regulatory strategy. What is the basis of strategic considerations, what are the considerations, what are the major components of a regulatory strategy, how do the different disciplines involved in drug development work together?

Table of Contents

4

1. LIST OF ABBREVIATIONS

ABDA	Arzneibüro Bundesvereinigung Deutscher Apothekerverbände
ADR	Adverse Drug Reaction
AE	Adverse Event
Afssaps	L'Agence française de sécurité sanitaire des produits de santé
AMIS	Arzneimittelinformationssystem
ATC	Anatomic, therapeutic chemical classification
BfArM	Bundesinstitut für Arzneimittel und Medizinprodukte
CADREAC	Collaboration Agreement between Drug Regulatory Agencies in EU Associated Countries
CDER	Center for Drug Evaluation and Research
CMC	Quality, Control, Manufacture
CMS	Concerned Member State
CPMP	Committee for Proprietary Medicinal Products
CTD	Common Technical Document
DGRA	Deutsche Gesellschaft für Regulatory Affairs
DIA	Drug Information Association
DIMDI	Deutsches Institut für Medizinische Dokumentation und Information
DPI	Dry Powder Inhaler
(D)RA	(Drug) Regulatory Affairs
eCTD	electronic Common Technical Document
EFTA	European Free Trade Association
EMC	Electronic medicines compendium
EMEA	European Agency for the Evaluation of Medicinal Products
EFPIA	European Federation of Pharmaceutical Industries and Associations
EPAR	European Public Assessment Report
EphMRA	European Pharmaceutical Market Research Association
FDA	Food and Drug Administration
FDAMA	Food and Drug Modernisation Act
FDC&A	Federal Food, Drug and Cosmetic Act
FOI	Freedom of Information
GxP	Good Practice in different areas (symbolised by the x)
HA	Health Authority
IFPMA	International Federation of Pharmaceutical Manufacturers Association
ICH	International Conference on Harmonisation of Technical Requirements
IMPD	Investigational Medicinal Product Dossier
IMS	Institute for Medical Statistics
IND	Investigational New Drug Application
INN	International non-proprietary name
ISE	Integrated Summary of Efficacy
ISS	Integrated Summary of Safety
JPMA	Japanese Pharmaceutical Manufacturers Association
MHLW	Ministry of Health, Labour and Welfare
MPA	Medical Products Agency
MRI	Mutual Recognition Index
MRP	Mutual Recognition Procedure
NDA	New Drug Application
NME	New Medical Entity
NIHS	National Institute of Health Service
NPV	Net Present Value
od	once daily

OPSR	Organisation for Pharmaceutical Safety and Research
PDR	Physician's Desk Reference
PhRMA	Pharmaceutical Research and Manufacturers of America
PDUFA	Prescription Drug User Fee Act
PERF	Pan European Regulatory Forum
PI	Package Insert
PMSB	Pharmaceutical and Medical Safety Bureau
PMDEC	Pharmaceuticals and Medical Devices Evaluation Center
RA	Regulatory Affairs
RAJ	Regulatory Affairs Journal
RMS	Reference Member State
ROI	Return-on-Investment
SBA	Summary Basis of Approval
SmPC	Summary Product Characteristics
SPC	Supplementory Protection Certificate
SNDA	Supplemental New Drug Application
URL	Uniform Resource Locater
USA	United States of America
tid	ter in die (three times a day)
VFA	Verband forschender Arzneimittelhersteller
WHO	World Health Organisation

2.　INTRODUCTION

Many disciplines claim "intelligence" as part of their business, e.g. marketing intelligence, business intelligence, regulatory intelligence. This document focuses on regulatory intelligence as a pre-requisite of the regulatory strategy for drug development until submission. Drug life cycle management after drug approval as well as aspects of generic drugs are not considered.

Today, there are many drugs for similar indications in the market (e.g. more than 20 beta-blockers for hypertension) and heavy financial constraints press the international health care systems. That means a restricted chance of reimbursement for new drugs in the market place that do not represent a really new therapeutic concept. In addition, increasing regulatory requirements before getting a drug approved by the authorities lead to more expensive programs for drugs under development. For all these reasons, the return-on-investment (ROI) decreases for newly developed drugs and companies no longer have resources, in terms of man power and money for drug research and drug development „by chance". Innovative, successful and financially reasonable drug research and development ("claims driven research and development") becomes more and more important. Pressure on the companies regarding „hit rate" for the transition of development candidates to marketed products and the time to market increases. Companies develop strategies on various levels of management in order to focus on promising projects in promising markets to make optimal use of the available resources and maximise the ROI. The general management defines indications of interest (strategic decision based on business intelligence) that the company is going to focus on. Background for the decision may be the unmet medical need, the potential market size and the resulting potential positive ROI (e.g. positive net present value [NPV] as a basis of calculation). This strategic decision is the rationale for research to focus on these indications. Once, research and basic screening is successfully done, drug development starts. Within this process, Regulatory Affairs takes a key role and supports the process of drug research and development over the entire development cycle.

One of the major Regulatory Affairs contributions to the overall drug development is the regulatory strategy for the development candidate. Regulatory intelligence is the basis for any strategic considerations within the regulatory department. Regulatory intelligence consists of the following key components:
- Competitor Information
- Regulatory Environment
- Legal Requirements.

At the start of drug development, the intelligence work, as part of the regulatory strategy, is initiated and needs to be refined and updated over the entire life cycle of the product including the pre-submission as well as post-submission phases.

3. COMPONENTS OF REGULATORY INTELLIGENCE

4.13.1 Competitor Information

Analysis of competitor information is one of the main components of a regulatory strategy. It is very helpful to know which important competitors are in the therapeutic area, the status of the competitive drug (pre-clinical, clinical phase, launched, where launched, post-approval commitments, ...), etc. There are various data sources of very different quality available depending on the region / country and product class of interest. Competitors evaluated should cover all stages of development. Of course, the contribution of Regulatory Affairs is greater in later stages of the drug development (e.g. little contribution to compounds in research, major contribution to compounds already registered).

3.1.1 Criteria for the definition of relevant competitors

The relevant competitors are usually defined in close co-operation with other disciplines. Important disciplines in this regard are the Medical and Marketing Departments. The Medical Department provides unique insights on the medical needs in the community, the "gold standard of therapy" for the target indication in the target region / country (e.g. inhaled glucocorticosteroids at higher doses plus a long acting inhaled β2-agonist twice daily for severe persistent asthma [1]). The Marketing department's contributions are more oriented towards market share of drugs already available in the market place, expected market share of drugs under development, market size, financial power of the market. Regulatory aspects for the choice of a competitor for analysis are mainly:

- Same area of indication
- Same mode of application (e.g. most recent approvals of Dry Powder Inhalers [DPIs])
- Pharmacovigilance aspects (e.g. other drugs with QT prolongation in case the development candidate shows QT effects)
- Recent launches in the target regions / countries
- Subjects of advisory board meetings
- Recent Market Authorisation withdrawals / rejections
- Subjects to interesting special subgroups like orphan drug status or paediatric development programs

3.1.2 Essential information to be gathered about competitors

Competitor analyses are done from various perspectives and by various disciplines in order to achieve a comprehensive picture about the competitive situation for a certain indication in the target regions / countries. The ultimate goal is to learn from other companies' experiences in terms of success and failures of their drug development.

3.1.2.1 Trade name

Trade names can be different in different regions and countries. The assignment of a trade name depends on cultural and linguistic habits. In addition to this, trade names need to be distinguishable from similar trade names in the country in order to avoid confusion in the pharmacies. Therefore, it is essential to have an overview on existing trade names in the target region / country. If a company aims for one global trade name this name needs to be acceptable to all target countries with their national languages. If the name sounds acceptable for English speaking countries it may have an unacceptable meaning in other languages. An example is the Mitsubishi car "Pajero" which is acceptable in English but means a strong insult in Spanish. So, the overview on already existing trade names is a basis to think about potential own trade names.

3.1.2.2 International Non-proprietary Name (INN)

The WHO (http://www.who.int/medicines/organization/qsm/activities/qualityassurance/inn/orginn.shtml) has a constitutional mandate to develop, establish and promote international standards with respect to biological, pharmaceutical and similar products. In this context, the WHO is responsible for the approval procedure of INNs. Each INN is a unique name which is globally recognised and public property. It facilitates the identification of pharmaceutical substances or active pharmaceutical ingredients. The general idea is to have identical prefixes or suffixes for one drug class (e.g. –bactam for beta-lactamase inhibitors, gli- for sulfonamide hypoglcaemics) [2], [3], [4]. The rest of the INN can be chosen by the applicant, and of course this provides an opportunity to "burn" the INN into the customer's mind. On the other hand, after the end of the patent / data protection period generic companies will enter the market place and may use the INN as part of their brand name (e.g. ASS Ratiopharm). The INN being "burned" into people's minds would be a disadvantage for the originator once generic competitors enter the market place. Therefore, the choice of the INN is important, and an overview on the competitor situation helps in terms of positioning their own product.

3.1.2.3 Drug class

The drug class of a competitor is important in order assess the market situation and to get a link to the associated ATC code (http://www.whocc.no/atcddd/). The ATC code is assigned by the WHO in order to reflect the major properties of a compound. In the Anatomical Therapeutic Chemical (ATC) classification system, the drugs are divided into different groups according to the organ or system on which they act and their chemical, pharmacological and therapeutic properties.

Drugs are classified in groups at five different levels. The drugs belong to one of fourteen main groups (1st level), with one pharmacological/therapeutic subgroup (2nd level). The 3rd and 4th levels are chemical/pharmacological/therapeutic subgroups and the 5th level is the chemical substance. The 2nd, 3rd and 4th levels are often used to identify pharmacological subgroups.

In various countries, the ATC code assigned to a drug is important for reimbursement by the respective health care system once the drug is approved by the Health Authority. Therefore, it is important to think about the "strategy" to apply for a certain ATC code: can the WHO be convinced that this drug under discussion is the first representative of a new drug class (e.g. in the area of antibiotics) and therefore is suitable for reimbursement? Is the drug under discussion the first member of a new antibiotic subclass (e.g. Penems) and therefore suitable for reimbursement? In various European countries, the third level of the ATC code is regarded as the "magic limit" to define new and reimbursable drugs.

Proposed new ATC codes are published in print (WHO Drug Information Journal and WHO Pharmaceutical Newsletter) and in the Internet (www.whocc.nmd.no) and interested parties are allowed a deadline (period not specified) to comment / object. With no objections received, the new ATC code will be considered final.

Another similar, but independent classification system, is the EPhMRA (European Pharmaceutical Market Research Association) classification (http://www.ephmra.org/site_map.html). The EPhMRA is used world-wide e.g. by IMS (Institute for Medical Statistics) for market research statistics within the pharmaceutical industry. Often, the company internal marketing analysis is based on IMS data. An important point to note about the EPhMRA system is that products are classified, not molecules. "Product" is defined as a pack or unit that can be dispensed, prescribed, etc. The products are classified according to their main therapeutic indication. Each product is assigned to one category. There is no apportionment of sales by usage, such as diagnosis value.

In the 1970s, WHO adapted the EPhMRA system for its own needs. This became the system that the WHO calls the Anatomical Therapeutic Chemical system (ATC). At the present time, the two systems are similar but are designed to meet two different goals. The purpose of the WHO ATC is to meet the needs of teaching, clinical trials, health organisations, and governments. The EPhMRA Anatomical Classification system must meet the needs of marketing research and marketing. The WHO ATC classifies substances while the EPhMRA/PBIRG Anatomical Classification system classifies products.

3.1.2.4   Type of Procedure

This aspect is mainly relevant for Europe. In Europe, three major types of approval procedures can be distinguished: the centralised procedure, the Mutual Recognition Procedure (MRP) and the purely national procedure (possible only in case of "one-country-submissions"). Each of the procedures has certain advantages and disadvantages.

The centralised procedure for authorising biotechnology-derived (mandatory) and highly innovative (by choice) medicines is laid down in Council Regulation (EEC) No 2309/93 [5]. The centralised procedure, which came into operation in 1995, allows applicants to obtain a marketing authorisation that is valid throughout the EU. When a company wishes to place a medicinal product that is eligible for the centralised procedure on the market, it submits an application directly to the EMEA (European Agency for the Evaluation of Medicinal Products), to be assessed by the Committee for Proprietary Medicinal Products (CPMP). Once the evaluation is completed, the CPMP gives a favourable or unfavourable opinion as to whether to grant the authorisation or not. The time limit for the evaluation procedure is 210 days, and the various steps during these 210 days are clearly defined. The Agency then has 30 days to forward its opinion to the Commission. This is the start of the second phase of the procedure: the decision-making process. The Agency sends its opinion to the Pharmaceutical Unit in the eleven Community languages, with annexes containing:

*   The summary of product characteristics
*   The particulars of the manufacturing authorisation holder responsible for batch release
*   The particulars of and the manufacturer of the biological active substance and
*   The conditions of the marketing authorisation
*   The labelling and the package leaflet.

During the decision-making process, the Commission services check marketing authorisation compliance with Community law and turn the Agency opinion into a binding decision for all the Member States. The Commission has 30 days to prepare a draft decision. The medicinal product is assigned to a Community registration number, which will be placed on its packaging if the marketing authorisation is granted. During this period, various Commission directorates-general are consulted on the draft marketing authorisation decision. They have 10 days to deliver their opinions [6] (http://pharmacos.eudra.org/F2/pharmacos/docs/brochure/pharmaeu.pdf). Centrally-authorised products may be marketed in all Member States.

Arrangements for implementing the mutual recognition procedure are laid down in Council Directive 2001/83/EC [10]. To be eligible for this procedure, a medicinal product must already have been authorised for marketing in one Member State. Since 1 January 1998, the mutual recognition procedure has been compulsory for all medicinal products to be marketed in a Member State other than that in which they were first authorised. Any national marketing authorisation granted by an EU Member State's national authority can be used to support an application for its mutual recognition by other Member States. The mutual recognition procedure works on the principle of the mutual recognition by EU Member States of their respective national marketing authorisations. An application for recognition may be addressed to one or more Member States. The applications submitted must be identical and all concerned Member States must be notified. The first country that evaluates the medicinal product via national procedure becomes the "Reference Member State" (RMS). It notifies this decision to other Member States ("Concerned Member States" [CMS]), to whom applications have also been submitted. CMS may then suspend their own evaluations, and await the RMS's detailed assessment report on the product. As soon as the assessment is completed, copies of this report are sent to all Member States and they then have 90 days to recognise the decision of the RMS and the SmPC as approved (by granting a marketing authorisations with identical SmPCs). In case any CMS refuses to recognise the original RMS national authorisation, e.g. on public health reasons, the reasons are submitted to the appropriate EMEA scientific committee (CPMP), for arbitration. The EMEA committee opinion is then forwarded to the Commission, for the start of the decision making process. As in the centralised procedure, this process entails consulting various Commission directorates-general and the regulatory standing committees on human medicinal products, as appropriate. Once the Commission decision is taken, it is binding for all the Member States concerned, which must withdraw, grant, or vary the marketing authorisations as necessary to comply with the decision. Other Member States not directly concerned at the time of the decision are also bound as soon as they receive a marketing authorisation application for the same product. In the event of a serious disagreement among Member States, which makes it impossible for the Commission to decide, a decision may be taken by the Council of the European Union [6]. The MRP can be repeated in order to include Member States that have not participated in the "first wave" of applications (repeat use of MRP).

A purely national application within the EU is only possible if the product under discussion is designated for being launched in one country only. This approach today is unusual as drug development usually does not focus on one single country. This purely national approach needs to be differenciated from the MRP approach that has the national approval in the RMS as a prerequisite.

Another differenciation of dossiers is "original dossier" and "line extension" (Europe) or sNDA (USA) (supplemental NDA).

This thesis only covers new medical or chemical entities until submission; generic applications as well as medical devices are excluded. Therefore, aNDA (abbreviated applications), sNDA etc. are not considered, only the submission of "original" dossiers.

3.1.2.5 Countries and the associated Submission date / Approval date

The overview of submission dates per country is an important source of information in order to get an idea about the competitor's submission strategy as well as authority driven hurdles. Example: if the competitor launched an antibiotic drug first in the USA, then in Germany and after Germany in Italy, Spain and Portugal at the same time and after that in many Asian countries the conclusion may be that the USA is the most important market for the company and FDA the most relevant authority that shows the way to future approvals in other countries. In Europe, the company probably chose a MRP with Germany as reference member state. As there are only "smaller" CMS (in terms of sales), there certainly is an issue in the dossier that led the company to the decision of not submitting (or withdrawing the dossier) in countries like France that represents a huge European antibiotic market and a very "difficult to handle" authority. After Europe, other markets have been discovered and entered. This conclusion can become relevant when developing the own submission strategy.

If in Europe a specific country shows up frequently as RMS or rapporteur for a specific drug class one may conclude that this agency has a certain experience in this indication area. Recent submissions in a country are a good hint for up-to-date knowledge of the agency for a specific area of indication. The delay between submission date (if accessible) and approval date gives an idea about the approval time in this country.

3.1.2.6 Clinical trials presented in the dossier

Clinical trials are an excellent source of competitive information as they are designed to reflect the future treatment situation / intention / positioning in the market. Most relevant pieces of information for analysis are the following:
- Inclusion / Exclusion criteria
- Indication

11

- Therapeutic regimen (first line, second line, ...)
- Trial design:
  - Controlled / uncontrolled trials
  - Parallel groups / crossover design
  - Number of treatment arms / crossover phases
  - Competitor
  - Co-medication (if relevant)
- Number of patients
- Countries involved
- Clinical endpoints
- Interactions with other drugs / food
- Studies in special populations, e.g.:
  - Hepatic / renal dysfunction
  - Elderly / paediatric patients / pregnant women
- Clinical trials initiated due to a post-approval commitment

For details refer to ICH guidance documents E6, E8, E10 (http://www.ich.org/UrlGrpServer.jser?@_ID=276&@_TEMPLATE=254).

3.1.2.7 Competitor labelling

In case the competitive compound is already in the market place, the approved SmPC / PI is absolutely helpful and allows comparisons between products in a country and between countries for one specific product. An interesting finding may be the non-mentioning of gonorrhoea for an antibiotic drug, and the explanation can be "not approved due to insufficient data" but may also be covered by the more general indication of "urinary tract infections". There may be countries with more explicit indications in their labelling (e.g. USA) and others with less explicit indications (e.g. Spain) which does not at all reflect properties of the product under evaluation but just country specific attitudes. These two aspects need to be distinguished from each other when evaluating national SmPCs. The differences between countries also need to be reflected when the appropriate European procedure is selected (MRP with RMS / CMSs, centralised procedure with rapporteur / co-rapporteur). In addition to the already mentioned national differences, one needs to keep in mind the regional difference, e.g. the US labelling is very different from the European SmPCs / PIs in terms of presentation and level of detail, and in the USA the patient information leaflet often is not provided to the patients (e.g. number of leaflets attached to the bottle insufficient or pharmacist does not print the patient related information out).

3.1.3 Sources of Competitor Information

3.1.3.1 Authority Homepages

In this section very few agency homepages are presented as examples for the type of information to be gathered from agency homepages.

3.1.3.1.1 FDA

The FDA homepage (www.fda.gov) is very helpful. One "room" within this homepage is the "Center for Drug Evaluation and Research" (CDER) (www.fda.gov/cder) which is dedicated to human drugs. The orange book (one link from the CDER homepage) contains all approved drug products in the USA and allows access to basic patent data, mainly patent number and patent expiration as well as basic information about the drug itself (applicant, approval date, ...). The link to "Drug Approvals" allows access to important information (Product name, Company, Application number, Approval Date, Letter Posted, Label Posted, Review Posted). In the optimal case, all these categories contain attached PDF-files. If these files are not posted the Summary Basis of Approval (SBA) can be requested from the FDA as paper copy. The information provided by the FDA is comprehensive and allows detailed conclusions about documentation provided to the FDA, the strengths and weaknesses of the dossier and that leads to "lessons learned" for the own development candidate. The National code directory (http://www.fda.gov/cder/ndc/database/default.htm) also provides brief tabulated information about the drug under discussion. Rationale for the provision of all the key information to the interested public is the "Freedom of Information Act" (FOI).

The FDA Advisory Committee homepage (www.fdaadvisorycommittee.com/FDC/AdvisoryCommittee/TOC.htm) provides alerts about the future sessions and results of the past advisory board meetings. The newsletter service can be ordered for free and keeps the Regulatory Affairs Manager always up-to-date with regard to the topics currently under discussion within the FDA. Given the appropriate IT equipment one is able to participate in the meetings via webcast. This allows even better information as one sees interactions between the meeting participants.

The MedWatch (www.fda.gov/medwatch/SAFETY/2002/safety02.htm#premar) represents the FDA safety information and adverse event reporting program and is a sound source of information about product-related and class-related safety issues. MedWatch also offers an E-mail alerting service for free.

3.1.3.1.2   EMEA

The European Public Assessment Report (EPAR) (http://www.emea.eu.int/htms/human/epar/epar.htm#) reflects the scientific conclusion reached by the Committee for Proprietary Medicinal Products (CPMP) at the end of the centralised evaluation process and provides a summary of the reasons for the CPMP opinion in favour or not in favour of granting a marketing authorisation for a specific medicinal product. It is made available by the EMEA (http://www.emea.eu.int) for information to the public, after deletion of commercially confidential information. The legal basis for its creation and availability is contained in Article 12 (4) of Council Regulation (EEC) No. 2309/93 [5]. The EPAR is a concise document which highlights the main parts of the CPMP scientific discussion leading to the CPMP opinion. The content of the EPAR is derived from the various reports produced during the centralised evaluation procedure, resulting from the review of the documentation submitted by the applicant, together with the scientific discussion at CPMP meetings. The EPAR is updated throughout the authorisation period as changes to the original terms and conditions of the authorisation (i.e. variations, pharmacovigilance issues, specific obligations) are made. The abstract, authorised presentations and the Commission Decision product information of all presentations are provided in all EU languages. The scientific discussion and procedural steps are available in English only.

The MRI Product Index (http://mri.medagencies.com/prodidx/) includes medicines approved in the Member States of the European Union according to the procedure for Mutual Recognition. The MRI contains at least information about RMS, CMSs, Marketing Authorisation Holder (MAH), MR-number, day 90 (for details see section 3.1.2.4). The more recent entries do also contain a link to the SmPC approved. If some of the information is missing, the solution would be to contact the RMS and ask for that piece of information.

The EMEA Web Site Map (http://www.emea.eu.int/sitemap.htm) links to various sections of the EMEA where interesting competitor information can be gathered (e.g. marketing authorisation withdrawals, press releases, referrals, pharmacovigilance opinions).

3.1.3.1.3   National European Health Authorities

The "Heads of Agencies" homepage (http://heads.medagencies.org/) links to the Health Agencies of all countries within the EU. Relevant national information as press releases and pharmacovigilance information can be picked up. Some agencies like the French L'Agence française de sécurité sanitaire des produits de santé (Afssaps) present their homepages in the national language only, other agencies like the Swedish Medicinal Products Agency (MPA) provide an English version of their homepage.

3.1.3.1.4   Japanese Health Authority

There are three Japanese Regulatory Authorities. One part of the "Ministry of Labor, Health and Welfare" (MLHW, Kosei Roudou Syo) is the Pharmaceutical and Medical Safety Bureau (PMSB) which finally approves a product. The Pharmaceuticals and Medical Devices Evaluation Center (PMDEC, Sinsa Senta) (http://www.mhlw.go.jp/english/) is part of the National Institute of Health Services (NIHS) and provides the evaluation of all dossiers (quality, efficacy and safety) for all prescription drugs and medical devices as well as proprietary drugs, quasi-drugs and cosmetics via an evaluation team. The Organisation for Pharmaceutical Safety and Research (OPSR, KIKO) provides consultation services to pharmaceutical companies (scientific advice), reviews the IND documents and checks GxP (Good Practice in different areas [symbolised by the x]) compliance.

Some of the URLs related to the Pharmaceuticals and Medical Devices Evaluation Center are provided in English, most of them are only available in Japanese language.

3.1.3.2   Company Homepages

In case the focus is on a specific product from a specific company one can access the company's homepage and gather information from there. Besides mainly product-related information (e.g. successful approval of product XYZ, the "top 10 products" of the company, overview of company's products), the companies' annual reports as well as the information sent out to shareholders and the agenda for the shareholder meetings are valuable sources of information.

3.1.3.3   Scientific Publications

Scientific publications can be obtained from journals like e.g. "British Medical Journal" (http://bmj.bmjjournals.com/). Many of these journals provide electronic versions that are accessible via the Internet. Focus of information gathered from these sources are published results of clinical studies, research results with new compounds, toxicological studies with compounds under development etc..

DIMDI (Deutsches Institut für Medizinische Dokumnetation und Information) (http://www.dimdi.de/de/db/index.htm) in Germany provides free of charge access to various scientific databases, including Medline and Cancerlit (Somed of limited relevance). Medline is one of the best known scientific databases in the medical field. Choosing appropriate search strategies, most of the medically relevant publications can be found in this database amongst them results of clinical studies in the area of indication under evaluation. If the number of patients within a trial is really huge and one product is an investigational product one might think about pivotal phase III trials necessary for a submission. The publication then is an essential source of information regarding study design and results.

Regulatory Affairs journals like RAJ (http://www.pjbpubs.com/cms.asp?pageid=875) provide information about Regulatory Affairs topics currently under discussion and potential regulations coming up in the mid-term future which might be important for the submission of the development candidate.

3.1.3.4   Scientific Internet Search Engines

iLOR (http://www.ilor.com/searchilor.lor?q=&searchselector=0), SCIRUS (http://www.scirus.com/) and PubMed (http://www.ncbi.nlm.nih.gov:80/entrez/query.fcgi?CMD=Add%20to%20Clipboard&DB=PubMed) are examples for scientific internet search engines. All of them have search algorithms in order to find the relevant publications. Level of up to dateness and relevance of the publications found need to be assessed. Many of the publications found are not free of charge except the abstract which often is enough to assess the relevance of the publication. As already mentioned in section 3.1.3.3 publications with a competitive compound are relevant in order to assess parts of the development plan of the competitive company.

3.1.3.5 General Internet Search Engines

This section briefly describes examples for search engines. No claim to completeness can be raised. Usually, it is helpful to refer to several search engines as their algorithms for calculating "relevance" of the documents found are different, and different documents are found. Relevant documents usually contain links to other documents and can therefore be regarded as the "starting point" for a new and more focussed search. The search engines presented in this section are "meta-search engines"; this means they cover a variety of other individual search engines which need not be addressed individually.

TABLE 1: EXAMPLES FOR INTERNET SEARCH ENGINES

Name of the Search Engine	Internet URL	Description
AltaVista	http://de.altavista.com/)	has a good search algorithm which also accepts boolean expressions and is a very valuable source of scientific information. Up to dateness and relevance need to be evaluated, but for some sample searches results of US advisory board meetings have been found which leads to the conclusion that the documents covered by this search engine can be relevant to Regulatory Affairs.
Google	(www.google.com)	is a very common search engine with many topics covered. Its value for this specific purpose is limited.
AllTheWeb	(http://www.alltheweb.com/search?query=&cat=web&type=all)	has a nice search engine with filters like "in text" "in title" that help to limit the documents found under a specific search item.
mamma	(http://www.mamma.com/)	is a valuable starting point for a web search and provides a valuable search algorithm.
Vivissimo	http://vivisimo.com/	is a valuable tool for literature research. Major strength is the clustering of documents according to an internal algorithm.

3.1.3.6 Labelling Databases

Labelling databases provide an overview on the currently marketed products and their SmPC and / or PI. Some labelling databases like the PDR (USA) provide extensive and very comprehensive information about all aspects of the product (CMC, pre-clinical investigations, clinical investigations) which allows many conclusions about the development program and study results of the competitor. Some of these data sources are free of charge (like the public section of the British eMC [Electronic medicines compendium]), others need to be paid before granting access (like the French Vidal). Most of these databases do not contain 100% of the products marketed in the respective country (e.g. Rote Liste in Germany).

Some examples for labelling databases are:

Country	Name of the database	Internet
Australia	MediMedia Austalia (MIMS)	http://www.mims.com.au/
Canada	Compendium Phamaceutical Specialties (CPS)	
France	Vidal	http://www.vidal.fr/
Finland	Pharmaca fennica	http://www.fennica.net/s/w/l/laakeopa.htm
Germany	Rote Liste, Gelbe Liste	www.rote-liste.de/
	ABDA database	www.gelbe-liste.de
	AMIS database	http://www.dimdi.de/de/db/recherche.htm
Japan	Japanese Pharmaceutical Reference (JPR)	http://www.e-search.ne.jp/~jpr/
Netherlands	Repertorium	
Sweden	FASS	http://www.fass.se/LIF/home/index.jsp
Switzerland	Arzneimittelkompendium der Schweiz	http://www.documed.ch/deutsch/
Spain	Vademecum International	http://vademecum.medicom.es/paginas_htm/FramesetPrincipal.asp
UK	Electronic Medicines Guide (eMC)	http://www.medicines.org.uk/
USA	Physician's Desk Reference (PDR)	http://www.pdr.net/pdrnet/librarian/action/command.Command
	Micromedex	

The German databases ABDA (Arzneibüro Bundesvereinigung Deutscher Apothekerverbände) and AMIS (Arzneimittelinformationssystem) are maintained and published by DIMDI (Deutsches Institut für Medizinische Dokumentation und Information) and provide detailed information about drugs in the German market.

4.23.2   Regulatory Environment

"Regulatory environment" means information from various sources which are not directly related to agency guidance documents.

3.2.1 Agency Benchmarks

Via internet, the available activity reports of various agencies offer more or less detailed overviews of drug applications / year. The agencies referred to in the following sections are meant as examples (major agencies with many applications per year. Japan has been excluded as no information could be found). Besides the benchmarking information, the agencies' activity reports provide insight in their general activities, in the focus of their work and allow conclusions about future development and future requests that may come up in these countries.

3.2.1.1   FDA

The last Food and Drug Administration's (FDA's) Center for Drug Evaluation and Research (CDER) „Report to the Nation 2002" (http://www.fda.gov/cder/reports/rtn/2002/RTN2002-1.HTM) gives a comprehensive drug review. In addition, approval times for NDAs and new molecular entities (NMEs) are available (see charts below).

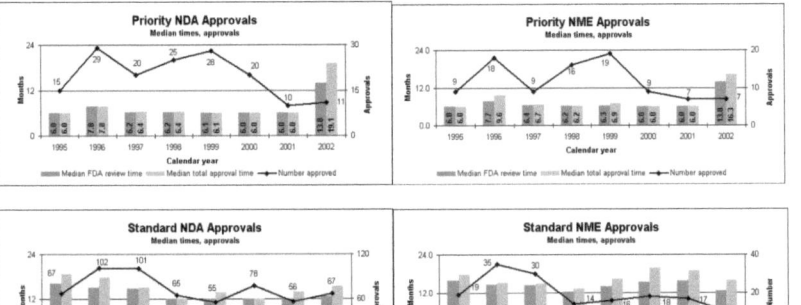

In 2002, a steep rise in median total approval times for priority NDAs and NMEs occured. According to the FDA, this was a statistical artefact caused by the approval of a number of older applications remaining from the 1999 and 2000 receipt cohort coupled with a significant decrease in the number of priority applications received in 2001 and 2002. With a smaller pool of recent priority applications with short approval times, the remaining "tail" of submissions for earlier years dominated the median approval time statistic.

Reasons for approval delays have been:
Standard NMEs:
- Safety issues (38 percent)
- Efficacy issues (21 percent)
- Manufacturing facility issues (14 percent)
- Labelling issues (14 percent)
- Chemistry, manufacturing, and controls issues (10 percent)
- Submission quality (3 percent)
Priority NMEs:
- Chemistry, manufacturing and controls issues (46 percent)
- Safety issues (27 percent)
- Efficacy issues (18 percent)
- Manufacturing facilities issues (9 percent)

This information can give interesting information for the own development candidate that is ready for submission. Safety seems to be the major concern for the FDA.

Applications for a new or expanded use, often representing important new treatment options, are formally called "efficacy supplements" to the original new drug application. The FDA has a goal of reviewing standard supplements in 10 months and priority supplements in six months. The new and expanded use review statistics on this page include figures for both priority and standard applications.

17

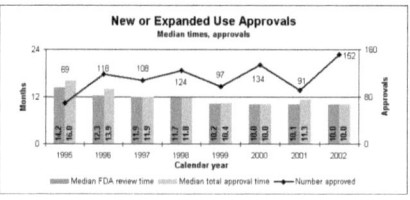

3.2.1.2   EMEA

The European Agency for the Evaluation of Medicinal Product (EMEA) published the Eighth Annual Report (2002) (http://www.emea.eu.int/pdfs/general/direct/emeaar/005502en.pdf) on their regulatory activities.

FIGURE 3: : APPROVAL TIMES FOR THE CENTRALISED PROCEDURE (SOURCE: 8TH ANNUAL REPORT 2002)

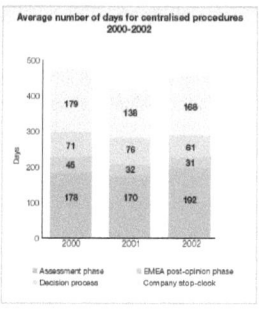

The overall assessment time slowed compared to 2001 due to the fact that there were no accelerated review procedures in 2002. In 2002, the EMEA introduced a simplified post opinion linguistic checking procedure with a view to reducing the administrative translation burden for both National Authorities and Industry. For procedural details please refer to section 3.1.2.4.

Corresponding information about the MRP is not very detailed. 587 new application have been submitted in 2002, 106 products have been under evaluation in 2002, 420 procedures ended positively in 2002, 2 referrals have been initiated.

3.2.1.3   Germany

The BfArM published the most recent data (January to November 2003) for Germany on their homepage (http://www.bfarm.de/de/Arzneimittel/statistik/stat-2003-internet.pdf), dated 12th and 15th of December 2003. No approval times are mentioned, only the number of applications per month. Reference is made to national as well as to European applications.

3.2.1.4   France

The Afssaps annual report 2002 (http://agmed.sante.gouv.fr/htm/5/indrap.htm) is only available in French language. Information about approval times is marginal although the authority activities are described in a very detailed and comprehensive way. The reader gets a clear picture of what the Afssaps did and plans to do. The median approval time increased from 159 days in 2001 to 213 days in 2002. As a consequence, the Afssaps reorganised the internal dossier review versus a centralised review within the agency independent from the mode of submission (national, MRP, centralised). Reference is made to national as well as to European procedures.

3.2.1.5   Conclusion

Based on the current agency activity reports, approval time for a "standard drug" would be similar in Europe and the USA and could be expected in the range of 15 and 18 months.

3.2.2   Regulatory Precedents on Other Products

Before granting a marketing authorisation for a specific medicinal product, often a scientific evaluation is performed by the respective Advisory Committees. The summaries of the evaluation processes are published. One example is presented from Europe (CPMP) and USA (FDA). For details about the European procedures see also section 3.1.2.

KETEK® / LEVVIAX® contains the active substance telithromycin. The CPMP adopted a positive opinion in March 2001 recommending approval of the product in the EU in all presented indications (community-acquired pneumonia, acute exacerbation of chronic bronchitis, acute sinusitis, and tonsillitis/pharyngitis caused by Group A *beta streptococci*.). In contrast, on 26 April 2001 the FDA's Advisory Committee recommended a granting for marketing authorisation for KETEK® in the USA only for the treatment of community-acquired pneumonia in patients 18 years of age and older. The decision was based on the risk/benefit analysis of the efficacy and safety information presented by Aventis Pharma S.A. The Advisory Committee listed major safety concerns, insufficiently studied issues and insufficient clinical information on efficacy in the indications rejected. Additional clinical experience was needed to support the approval of KETEK® for the further two indications. Additional information from ongoing studies concerning the clinical efficacy of KETEK® against resistant strains of *S. pneumoniae* should be provided. The fourth indication was not even addressed because tonsillitis/pharyngitis is a mild disease, and the target population is typically the paediatric population. Aventis Pharma S.A.'s application included data from patients 13 years of age and older. The recommendation of the FDA's Advisory Committee was limited to one indication although the same data were filed for application in the USA and in Europe [7], [8], [9].

It is obvious that a thoroughly proven efficacy for each single indication and a rigid clinical safety evaluation are major issues for marketing authorisations. Different authorities look differently at data, and it is helpful to have precedents in place in order to find out during the planning phase of the clinical program which pre-requisites need to be fulfilled. This helps to get approval for all the indications studied. The conclusion from the example would be to plan the clinical studies for acute exacerbation of chronic bronchitis, acute sinusitis as well as tonsillitis/pharyngitis differently and ask for a scientific advice or pre-phase-III meeting with the FDA before starting the clinical program in order to improve the chances for an US approval.

Another source for knowledge based on the submission of precedents are company-internal precedents. The company has in-depth knowledge about the development, the authority discussions as well as the deficiency letters from the various authorities during the approval process which can be used as a "lesson learnt".

3.2.3   Ongoing and Future Regulatory Changes

Future Regulatory changes should be carefully followed up in order to make sure that the future dossier for the development candidate will fulfil the regulatory requirements of that future point in time. Some examples for changes in Europe and within the ICH region are presented in the following sub-sections.

3.2.3.1   Review 2001 (Europe)

The Regulatory Review 2001 foresees the following legislative and procedural changes:

- The CTD has to be used for all marketing authorisation applications (for details please refer to section 3.2.3.4)
- The name of the EMEA will be simplified into „European Medicines Agency" and of the CPMP will change into „Committee for Medicinal Products for Human Use"
- The CPMP will consist of only one expert from each member state instead of two
- In addition to biotechnological products the centralised procedure will be mandatory for new chemical entities intended to treat AIDS, cancer, neurodegenerative disorders or diabetes mellitus.
- Establishment of an „accelerated assessment procedure" for drugs suggesting a high therapeutic benefit
- First marketing authorisation will be valid for 5 years only. Application for extension of the registration needs to be made six months before the end of the period at the latest. If extension is granted by the competent authority, second registration will be valid for an undefined period. This means no renewal procedures will be performed
- Any marketing authorisation not followed by placing the drug on the market within the first 3 years will cease to be valid automatically
- Establishment of a European pharmacovigilance system including a database and an information transfer network between the European Health Authorities.

3.2.3.2   EU Enlargement

From 1st of May 2004 onwards, the EU will have 10 new member states: Czech Republic, Poland, Cyprus, Estonia, Hungary, Latvia, Lithuania, Malta, Slovakia and Slovenia. The political criterion for "joining the club" has been the stability of institutions guaranteeing democracy, human rights and the respect for minorities. The economic criterion has been the existence of a well working market economy. The regulatory criterion has been the "regulatory acquis criterion": the candidate countries must agree to bring their laws into compliance with the Acquis communautaire (body of the EU law) by the time of accession. Tools initiated by the EU to facilitate a smooth expansion of the EU pharmaceutical market are PERF (pan European Regulatory Forum) (http://perf.eudra.org/) and CADREAC (collaboration agreement between drug regulatory agencies in EU associated countries) (http://www.cadreac.org/content.htm). PERF tries to help the candidate countries to fulfil the requirements of the Acquis communautaire in respect of the pharmaceutical sector as preparation for their EU accession. PERF is mainly an inter-agency training effort. Current focus is the upgrade of old dossiers and the phasing-in. R&D industry is invited to provide programmatic proposals for phasing-in issues. CADREAC aims to facilitate the smooth transition of regulatory conditions in candidate countries to reach the EU regulatory standards. This includes the development of simplified procedures for granting marketing authorisations in the candidate countries for products authorised via centralised procedure / MRP in the EU. For centrally authorised EU-products, the central authorisation supersedes the national application, and no upgrading of the dossier is necessary. For MRP EU-products, the dossier has to be upgraded in case it does not yet comply with EU requirements. For this purpose, one can rely on existing and approved EU dossiers; recent renewals are particularly helpful. For all other products that are the "same" as products nationally authorised in the EU upgrading is necessary. The candidate country's assessment of a dossier submitted can be based on the EU dossier, detailed requirements for such dossiers are published by some candidate countries. Generic products can reference to a product with a self-standing dossier that complies with the Acquis and for which any data protection period has expired. For some cases one will not find the reference product in the local market, in that case reference to well-established- use is recommended (if possible) (http://www.emea.eu.int/euenlargement.htm).

These roughly described procedures during the transition phase towards the EU accession require thorough attention and follow-up as the accession process is dynamic, rules change, get more detailed, other companies gain experience that may be a "lesson learned" for the own company, the candidate countries establish new regulations based on first experiences and so on.

3.2.3.3 Implementation of the Clinical Trial directive (Directive 2001/20/EC)

This section is mainly taken from the EMEA page (http://www.emea.eu.int/Inspections/GCPgeneral.html).

Europe has adopted the ICH-GCP (http://www.ich.org/UrlGrpServer.jser?@_ID=276&@_TEMPLATE=254) guideline in July 1996. Now, it has been transferred to a legally binding directive which is published in EudraLex Volume 1 (http://pharmacos.eudra.org/F2/eudralex/vol-1/home.htm). Good Clinical Practice (GCP) is an international ethical and scientific quality standard for designing, recording and reporting trials that involve the participation of human subjects. Compliance with this standard provides public assurance that the rights, safety and well being of trial subjects are protected, consistent with the principles that have their origin in the Declaration of Helsinki, and that the clinical trial data are credible. Clinical trials included in any marketing authorisation application in the EU are required by Directive 2001/83/EC Annex I [10] to be conducted in accordance with GCP.

Requirements for the conduct of clinical trials in Europe including GCP and GMP and inspections of these, have been implemented in the Clinical Trial Directive (Directive 2001/20/EC) [11]. Information concerning the activities in Member States can be found via the Heads of Agencies web site. Implementation of the directive into local legislation has to be finished by 1st of May, 2004. National implementation of a directive may be adopted to national peculiarities without changing the overall meaning. Information concerning most candidate countries for EU membership can be found at the CADREAC web site (http://www.cadreac.org/content.htm). The implementation of the directive is not yet finished and needs careful monitoring regarding timing and implementation in the various countries. In Germany, the 12th amendment of the German Drug Law is under preparation and will include the implementation of the clinical trial directive. Development, implementation and implications of this 12th revision of the German Drug Law need careful follow-up.

Important topics for pharmaceutical companies are:
- Applications to Ethics Committee
- Valid request for authorisation to the competent authority, amendments, declaration of end of trial (IMPD)
- Clinical trial database (Eudract)
- Adverse events reports
- To be applied for "commercial" (industry) and "non-commercial" (e.g. physicians, academia) studies

This directive has a major impact on the planning of clinical programs, mainly on time and the amount of documentation that needs to be provided to the authority in order to get the permission to start a clinical trial. Until now, in Germany a limited amount of documentation needed to go into the BfArM-Vorlage. After the 1st of May, 2004 the complete IMPD needs to be provided, and until now, no clear guidance has been published by the BfArM. These facts need to be reflected in the regulatory strategy and the regulatory contributions to the clinical development plan.

3.2.3.4 Implementation of the CTD structure for Dossiers

The CTD is a global initiative across region level submissions within the ICH realm (ICH M4 [12]). It creates a harmonised approach to the submission format, which is expected to be more cost effective and efficient than the former regional / local approaches. The global authorities will review a (ideally identical) core set of data, which will help achieve consistent labelling world-wide. One needs to keep in mind that the possible dossier content is not at all concerned by this approach; harmonisation of the guidelines setting the requirements for the content will remain a major global challenge. The CTD format is mandatory since 1st of July, 2003 in Europe, Japan and Canada. In Switzerland, the CTD format is mandatory since 1st of January 2004. The USA highly recommend the CTD format since July 1st, 2003. The scope of the CTD format is as in table 3.

TABLE 3: SCOPE OF THE CTD FORMAT

	EU	FDA	MHLW
New chemical entities	included	included	included
New biologic	included	included*	included
New indication	included	included	included
New dosage forms	included	included	included
New route of administration	included	included	included
Generics/ OTC	included	included	not included
Variations/ SNDAs	included	included	included

* with the exception of blood and blood components

The CTD follows a 5 module approach with designated areas for regional specific information.

FIGURE 4: CTD STRUCTURE

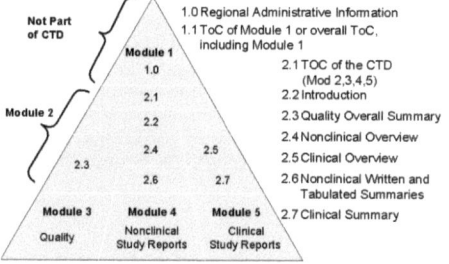

The regional / local information (module 1) is not harmonised. There is a certain danger that module 1 might become the thrashdump for all the special national requirements like the US ISS / ISE or the Japanese Gayo. The Regulatory Affairs Manager needs to monitor carefully new requests and guidance from various agencies including ICH regarding the CTD format.

The ICH M4 Expert Working Group (EWG) has defined the Common Technical Document (CTD). The ICH M2 Expert Working Group has defined the specification for the Electronic Common Technical Document (eCTD). The eCTD is defined as an interface for industry to agency transfer of regulatory information while at the same time taking into consideration the facilitation of the creation, review, lifecycle management and archival of the electronic submission. The specification for the eCTD is based upon content defined within the CTD. The CTD describes the organisation of modules, sections and documents. The structure and level of detail specified in the CTD have been used as the basis for defining the eCTD structure and content but where appropriate, additional details have been developed within the eCTD specification. Open standards, including proprietary standards, which through their widespread use can be considered de facto standards, are deemed to be appropriate [13] (http://www.ich.org/MediaServer.jser?@_ID=563&@_MODE=GLB).

EU Authorities accept the eCTD; however for legal reasons limited numbers of paper copies are required. Japan's legal copy is paper and electronic submissions are looked at case by case. The

FDA accepted electronic NDAs and therefore will accept a CTD in electronic format. Canada accepts Word Perfect and PDF files with a limited number of paper copies.

Benefits of electronic submissions are:
- Allow for the sharing of internal resources globally in the submission authoring and compilation
- Faster review which can be conducted globally
- More efficient archiving
- Faster to respond to internal / authority questions

3.2.4 Trade Associations

There are trade associations on a global, regional and national basis. Trade associations represent the opinion of their members and are in close discussion with the industry and the agencies and should therefore be recognised as part of the regulatory environment. They often collect comments on new guidance documents so that one can get an idea on the current thinking within the pharmaceutical industry, the regulatory agencies and the health care systems. Trade associations are also a vehicle to publish research results (e.g. VFA publishes on its homepage "breast cancer study cancelled due to obvious efficacy") and provide a useful source of information. The following sub-sections provide some examples of trade associations.

3.2.4.1   VFA

The (http://www.vfa.de/) is a German trade association and represents the researching pharmaceutical industry. The VFA focuses on the German health system (in particular providing patients with innovative drugs, making the health care system affordable for all citizens) and improving the conditions for research oriented pharmaceutical industry in Germany. The VFA is also a publication medium for various kinds of information (e.g. results of clinical studies, health care programs).

3.2.4.2   EFPIA

The European Trade association EFPIA (http://www.efpia.org/1_efpia/mission.htm) is situated in Brussels and has, as its members, Member Associations in sixteen countries in Western Europe. Much of the Federation's work is concerned with the activities of the European Commission and the EMEA. Companies in membership of EFPIA are manufacturers of prescription medicines and include all of Europe's major research-based pharmaceutical companies. A wide network of experts and country coordinators has been established, through Member Associations, to ensure that EFPIA's views within ICH represent the European industry. The EFPIA's main policy objectives are:
- To improve European healthcare market environment - in Europe today and an enlarged Europe tomorrow
- To maintain high standards of intellectual property protection in Europe and world-wide
- To set up an efficient and high-quality system for the approval of medicines in Europe based on quality, safety and efficacy, which ensures that new medicines reach patients rapidly.

The EFPIA publishes comments on draft guidance documents and represents the "European voice" in global environments.

3.2.4.3   JPMA

The Japanese trade association JPMA (http://www.jpma.or.jp/12english/index.html) represents 90 member companies. Membership includes all the major research-based pharmaceutical manufacturers in Japan. Among the objectives of JPMA is the development of a competitive pharmaceutical industry with a greater awareness and understanding of international issues. JPMA promotes and encourages the adoption of international standards (e.g. ICH standards) by its member companies.

The JPMA is a voluntary organisation of research-based pharmaceutical manufacturers that contribute to society by developing new pharmaceuticals. Member companies maintain appropriate communications with the aims of promoting balanced public understanding of industry issues and finding solutions to such issues in order to support the sound development of the industry. The JPMA works in close co-operation with the International Federation of Pharmaceutical Manufacturers Associations (IFPMA).

3.2.4.4   PhRMA

The US trade association Pharmaceutical Research and Manufacturers of America (PhRMA) (http://www.phrma.org/) represents the research-based industry in the USA. The association has 67 companies in membership which are involved in the discovery, development and manufacture of prescription medicines. There are also 24 research affiliates which conduct biological research related to the development of drugs and vaccines.

3.2.4.5   IFPMA

The IFPMA (International Federation of Pharmaceutical Manufacturers Associations) (http://www.ifpma.org/) is a non-profit, non-governmental Organisation (NGO) with membership of the world-wide research-based pharmaceutical industry and manufacturers of prescribed medicines including developed and developing countries. In the research and development pipeline, the industry is working on more than 700 new medicines and vaccines for infectious diseases including HIV/AIDS, cancer, heart disease and stroke, and diseases that disproportionately affect women, such as osteoporosis.
The IFPMA has three primary tasks:
- Develop global position statements on matters of health care policy
- Encourage the global exchange of information within the industry
- Work closely with international organisations dedicated to health and trade-related issues, including the World Health Organisation, the World Bank, the World Trade Organisation and the World Intellectual Property Organisation and ICH (IFPMA runs the ICH Secretariat.)

3.2.5 Regulatory Associations

Some examples for regulatory associations are:
- AFAR (Association Francaise des Affaires Reglementaires) (http://www.afar.asso.fr/html/index.php)
- BIRA (British Institue of Regulatory Affairs) (http://www.bira.org.uk/Resource.phx/community/mainpage/mainpage.htx)
- DGRA (Deutsche Gesellschaft für Regulatory Affairs) (http://www.dgra.de/vorst/fr-vorst.htm)
- ESRA (European Society for Regulatory Affairs) (http://www.esra.org/Resource.phx/community/mainpage/mainpage.htx)

The ESRA homepage (http://www.esra.org/Resource.phx/public/resources/links.htx) provides a comprehensive overview on world-wide interesting links to agencies, health ministries, world-wide acting institutions like ICH, industry associations, pharmacopoeial commissions, health information sides etc.

The regulatory associations define themselves as being a neutral communication platform for the discussion between industry, agencies, universities, ministries and other bodies involved in the regulatory business. As the complexity of the Regulatory Affairs work increases constantly (e.g. new guidance documents, implications of the European enlargement, global initiatives) it becomes more and more important that Regulatory Affairs Managers are well trained and educated. Training of Regulatory Affairs Managers is another focus of the regulatory associations.

3.2.6 WHO

The World Health Organisation (WHO) (http://www.who.int/en/), the United Nations agency for health, was established on 7 April 1948. WHO's objective, as set out in its constitution, is the attainment of the highest possible level of health by all peoples. Health is defined in WHO's constitution as a state of complete physical, mental and social well-being and not merely the absence of disease or infirmity. WHO is governed by 192 Member States through the World Health Assembly. The Health Assembly is composed of representatives from WHO's Member States. The main tasks of the World Health Assembly are to approve the WHO programme and the budget for the following biennium and to decide major policy questions.

In carrying out its activities, WHO's secretariat focuses its work on the following 6 core functions:

* Articulating consistent, ethical and evidence-based policy and advocacy positions
* Managing information by assessing trends and comparing performance, setting the agenda for and stimulating research and development
* Catalysing change through technical and policy support, in ways that stimulate co-operation and action and help to build sustainable national and inter-country capacity
* Negotiating and sustaining national and global partnerships
* Setting, validating, monitoring and pursuing the proper implementation of norms and standards
* Stimulating the development and testing of new technologies, tools and guidelines for disease control, risk reduction, health care management, and service delivery

As the WHO is responsible for certain norms and standards it is important to carefully monitor their publications and discussions e.g. regarding ATC coding or "assessment and monitoring of antimalarial drug efficacy for the treatment of uncomplicated falciparum malaria" [14].

3.2.7 Training courses and Meetings

Interdisciplinary meetings like a Drug Information Association (DIA) annual meeting or training courses on specific Regulatory items, e.g. "How to compile a dossier based on the Common Technical Document (CTD) format" are good opportunities to get an idea on the thinking in the "Regulatory World" and the experiences of agencies and other companies.

3.3 Legal Requirements

The term „Legal Requirements" for the purpose of this document is defined as the supranational and authority requirements for drugs under development in order to get approval. The general requirements are described in sub-section 3.3.1. Besides the general requirements for drug development and dossier generation, there are often specific guidelines available for certain areas of indication; section 3.3.2 gives an example. The sections thereafter describe as models some specific aspects that are relevant for many drug developments. The discussion of the orphan drug status is meant as an example for the strategic considerations of the positive and negative aspects of a specific opportunity.

Of course, each development candidate has its peculiarities (e.g. chirality, liposome formulation, inherent Qt-issues, specific patient sub-populations like renally impaired patients or paediatric patients) which need to be handled, and special guidance documents valid for the region of interest need to be looked for.

3.3.1 General Requirements

3.3.1.1   Supra-national Guidance - Example: ICH
This section is mainly taken from the Internet information provided by the ICH (http://www.ich.org/UrlGrpServer.jser?@_ID=276&@_TEMPLATE=254).

The International Conference on Harmonisation of Technical Requirements for Registration of Pharmaceuticals for Human Use (ICH) is a unique project that brings together the regulatory authorities of Europe, Japan and the United States and experts from the pharmaceutical industry in the three regions (represented by the trade associations EFPIA, JPMA, PhRMA) to discuss scientific and technical aspects of product registration. The purpose is to make recommendations on how to achieve greater harmonisation in the interpretation and application of technical guidelines and requirements for product registration in order to reduce or obviate the need to duplicate the testing carried out during the research and development of new medicines. The focus of ICH is on the technical requirements for medicinal products containing new drugs. Since ICH was initiated, in 1990, there have been observers to act as a link with non-ICH countries and regions. The observers to ICH are:

- The World Health Organisation (WHO)
- The European Free Trade Association (EFTA), represented at ICH by Switzerland
- Canada, represented at ICH by Health Canada

The CADREAC countries accept the results of ICH activities.

The ICH does not develop legally binding guidance documents, but its activities reflect the current state of the art and the "burning issues". Many of the ICH guidance documents are transferred into local regulations with a certain delay.

One example is the ICH M4 "CTD" [12]. This guideline has been developed by the ICH and adopted to national law with the original wording (e.g. Europe: Notice to Applicants). For details see section 3.2.3.4.

Another recent example is the ICH harmonised tripartite guideline E6 "Guideline for Good Clinical Practice" from 1st of May, 1996 [15]. This ICH guideline has been accepted by the CPMP in July 1996 with the wording of the ICH guideline and is applicable for Europe since 1997 without becoming legally binding at that point in time. It has been transferred into the European legislation via the Directive 2001/20/EC from 4th of April, 2001.[11]. The directive has to be included into the national legislation of all EU member states until 1st of May, 2004 (see also section 3.2.3.3). This example shows how the non-binding ICH guidelines come down into national law. Therefore, it is very advisable to follow up the ICH discussions in order to be prepared for changes of the national legislation triggered by the ICH process. Although ICH E6 has become legally binding in Europe, the USA published it in the "Federal Register" in May 1997, but there is no effort to make it part of the US legislation. Japan included the ICH E6 guideline as an addendum of the "Pharmaceutical Law" in 1997 which lead to dramatic changes in the way clinical research is done in Japan. Major changes of the Japanese clinical research are

- The patient has to sign off the informed consent
- Physicians have to follow study protocols generated by the sponsors
- Timelines for clinical studies are now comparable to US and EU standards

Until 1996, clinical trials in Japan have mainly been influenced by the interest of opinion leaders, and the sponsor had only restricted influence on the conduct of the studies. The results of clinical studies had to be published in official journals in order to be acceptable to the authority as part of a dossier.

Another interesting topic is the ICH E5 (Ethnic factors) [16] which leads more and more to the acceptance of foreign data in Japan. The traditional way of getting a marketing authorisation in Japan has been to perform a complete drug development program locally in Japan. Now, the Japanese authority goes the way of accepting more and more foreign data. The Japanese authority tends to request a bridging study in order to show that Japanese diet and Japanese metabolism are not different compared to non-Japanese patients. This is a major improvement in terms of drug development time and expenses, and it is important to carefully monitor the increasing application of ICH E5. One approach may be to perform PK/PD studies in Japanese as well as in non-Japanese patients. If no differences are seen Japanese patients become part of the global development plan. In future, the J-NDA will be submitted utilising results of Japanese and non-Japanese clinical studies.

These examples show that it is essential to monitor the ICH homepage and be aware of recent discussions, drafts of certain guidance documents in order to anticipate modifications of the "state of the art" and prepare the best documentation for a dossier.

3.3.1.2   Europe

The European Commission's Pharmaceutical Unit runs a variety of information and communication projects, collectively known as "Eudra" projects (http://pharmacos.eudra.org/F2/pharmacos/docs/brochure/pharmaeu.pdf), which harness the latest electronic communications technology to further the European Commission's public health and single market policy aims. One of the key "Eudra" projects is EudraLex – the Community Legislation. The Pharmaceutical Unit of the European Commission makes Community pharmaceutical legislation, guidelines, the Notice to Applicants and other relevant Community texts available on the web server (http://pharmacos.eudra.org/F2/eudralex/index.htm). The "notice to applicants" is available in EudraLex volume 2 and describes the European application procedures.

In general, in Europe there are three different procedures in order to get a Marketing Authorisation:
- MRP based on the Directive 2001/83/EC of the European Parliament and of the Council of 6 November 2001 on the Community Code relating to medicinal products for human use [10]
- Centralised Procedure based on the Council Regulation 2309/93/EEC of 22 July 1993 [5]
- National Marketing Authorisation based on the national legislation

For details see section 3.1.2.4.

The Regulatory Affairs Manager needs to be familiar with the current status of the European Regulations, Directives, Decisions, Guidelines, Points to Consider and Communications.

3.3.1.3   Japan

Pharmaceutical administration in Japan is based on various laws and regulations, consisting mainly of: (1) the Pharmaceutical Affairs Law, (2) the Pharmacists Law, (3) the law concerning the Organisation for Pharmaceutical Safety and Research, (4) the Blood Collection and Blood Donation Services Control Law, (5) the Poisonous and Deleterious Substances Control Law, (6) the Narcotics and Psychotropics Control Law, (7) Cannabis Control Law, (8) the Opium Law, and (9) the Stimulants Control Law. For the enforcement and management of these laws, detailed regulations are prepared by the MHLW (ministry for health, labour and welfare), (http://www.mhlw.go.jp/english/index.html) in the form of ministerial ordinances and notices, such as the Enforcement Ordinance and the Enforcement Regulations of the Pharmaceutical Affairs Law, and notifications issued by the Director General of the Bureau or the directors of the Divisions in charge in the Ministry of Health, Labour, and Welfare. Details are described in [17] (http://www.jpma.or.jp/12english/index.html, section Regulations)" and the appendix 2003 under the same Internet link. The English versions of these documents are published by the Japanese trade association JPMA.

27

3.3.1.4   USA

The legal basis for Regulatory Affairs is the Code of Federal Regulations (CFR) (http://www.gpoaccess.gov/cfr/about.html). CFR is the codification of the general and permanent rules published in the Federal Register by the executive departments and agencies of the Federal Government. It is divided into 50 titles that represent broad areas subject to Federal regulation. Each volume of the CFR is updated once yearly. Title 21 is reserved for rules of the FDA, updated on the 1st of April and needs to be adhered to for regulatory business.

The second basic justification for the FDA and related Regulatory Affairs activities is the Federal Food, Drug and Cosmetic Act (FDC&A) (http://www.fda.gov/opacom/laws/fdcact/fdctoc.htm). Chapter 2 provides definitions for concepts like "drug product, drug substance, abbreviated application" which are important for Regulatory Affairs, chapter 5 deals with drugs and devices in particular.

FDA guidance documents (http://www.fda.gov/ora/ora_home_page.html) are published for all areas of drug development and support the interaction between industry and the FDA. They represent the agency's current thinking on particular subjects and are not legally binding for the agency and the sponsor, but it is advisable to have a good reason in place for not following them.

The Division of Dockets Management (DM) (http://www.fda.gov/ohrms/dockets/default.htm), formerly known as Dockets Management Branch, serves as the official repository for the administrative proceedings and rule-making documents for the Food and Drug Administration (FDA), an operating division of the Department of Health and Human Services (HHS).

The Prescription Drug User Fee Act (PDUFA) (http://www.fda.gov/oc/pdufa/PDUFAIII Goals.html) and the Food and Drug Modernisation Act (FDAMA) (http://www.fda.gov/opacom/7modact.html) are other important US guidance documents to adhere to. In 1992, the US Congress passed the PDUFA which authorises the FDA to collect fees from companies that produce certain human drugs and biological products. The additional revenue allowed the FDA to hire more reviewers and support staff and upgrade its information technology to speed up the application review process. The FDAMA reauthorised the PDUFA and induced major drug legislation reforms.

3.3.1   Therapeutic Area Guidance – Example: Microbial Diseases

For many therapeutic areas, specific guidance is available from agencies as well as from medical societies (medical guidance usually provided by the medical expert and basis for the design of the clinical trials in terms of treatment regimen, competitor etc.). For this document, microbial diseases have been taken as an example.

Europe:
- CPMP "Note for Guidance on Evaluation of new anti-Bacterial Medicinal Products" has been released in May 2003 for consultation and is the most recent document available for this purpose [18]
- "Points to Consider on Pharmacokinetics and Pharmacodynamics in the Development of Antibacterial Medicinal Products" have been approved in July 2000 [19]
- "Concept paper on the development of the revision of the committee for the proprietary medicinal products (CPMP) note for guidance (NFG) on evaluation of new anti-bacterial medicinal products (CPMP/EWP/588/95) and the CPMP NFG on the pharmacodynamic sections of the SPC for anti-bacterial medicinal products (CPMP/EWP/520/96)" [20].

USA:
- "Developing Antimicrobial Drugs — General Considerations for Clinical Trials" has been issued in 1998 by the FDA and is the most recent guideline available for this purpose [21]

- "Clinical Development and Labelling of Anti-Infective Drug Products" has been issued in 1997 by the FDA [22].

3.3.2 Special Populations – Example: Paediatric Patients

Relevant guidance is provided by the following documents:
- ICH E11: Clinical investigation of medicinal products in the paediatric population
- FDA: Department of Health and Human Services: 21 CFR Parts 201, 312, 314 and 601 [Docket No. 02N-0152]: Obtaining timely paediatric studies of and adequate paediatric labeling for human drugs and biologicals
- FDA: Guidance for Industry: Qualifying for Pediatric Exclusivity under Section 505A of the Federal Food, Drug and Cosmetic Act
- FDA: General Considerations for Pediatric Pharmacokinetic Studies for Drugs and Biological Products (Issued 11/1998) ICH E11: Clinical investigation of medicinal products in the paediatric population
- FDA: Pediatric Equity Act, 3.12.2003
- Europe: CPMP "Note for Guidance on Clinical Investigation of Medicinal Products in Children" CPMP/EWP/462/95) – adopted March 97 and "Better Medicines for children" – issued 2002 by the European Commission.

The classification of age groups should be done according to the ICH guideline as follows:
Pre-term new-born infants
- Term new-born infants (0 to 27 days)
- Infants and toddlers (28 days to 23 months)
- Children (2 to 11 years)
- Adolescents (12 to 16-18 years)

The US and European Regulatory Authorities encourage the companies to perform specific studies in childhood, as children are no "small adults". The "paediatric rule" of the USA contains provision for industry-FDA meetings and early consultation during the investigational study in order to facilitate the design and timely conduct of adequate paediatric studies. The "paediatric rule" enables the FDA to require the development of a paediatric formulation from companies. The incentive for companies to invest into the relatively small paediatric market is a 6-month additional market exclusivity. In the USA, waiving of clinical studies in children in the NDA dossier requires justification.

Europe is not yet that far advanced in the area of studies in paediatric patients. The European Commission proposes regulatory actions on paediatric medicinal products. It is suggested to routinely require studies in paediatric populations as part of the Market Authorisation Application requirements. A European expert group for paediatric medicines, which would determine whether or not the studies were acceptable in compliance with Directive 2001/20/EC [11], would screen the trials performed. A central database shall be set up providing information on paediatric formulations. The implementation is expected within the next 4 years.

Agencies' awareness for the need of valid patient data in controlled paediatric studies increases heavily, and the way of argumentation has reversed, that means the company needs to explain why they do not perform a paediatric program instead of arguing why they should perform research in this vulnerable young patient group.

3.3.3 Orphan Drug Designation

Drugs intended for illnesses occurring only in small patients populations (e.g. in Europe: HIV patients, certain types of cancer, cystic fibrosis patients) are called „Orphan Drugs". As the patient groups are small and no major return on development investment can be expected the industry is reluctant in developing that kind of drug. On the other hand, there is a high medical need for innovative drugs e.g. for HIV patients, and many Health Authorities try to offer financial incentives in order to motivate the pharmaceutical industry.

Regulatory basis is provided in:

- the USA by:
  - Orphan Drug Act signed in 1983
  - 21 CFR Part 316 (57 FR 62076)
  - Tax Credit: Section 45C of the Internal Revenue Code (Public Law Sec. 604/105-34)
- the EU by:
  - Regulation No. 141/2000 of 16 December 1999 on Orphan Medicinal Products
  - Procedure for Orphan Medicinal Product Designation (EMEA/14222/00/Rev 2)
  - Commission Guideline on the format and content of applications for designation ... (ENTR/6283/00 Rev1)
  - Points to consider on the calculation and reporting of the prevalence of a condition for orphan designation (COMP/436/01)
  - Note for Guidance on the format and content of the Annual Report on the state of Development of an Orphan Medicinal Product (COMP/189/01)
- Australia by:
  - Amendment to Therapeutic Goods Regulation1990
  - Subregulation 16H: Orphan Drug (Part 3B definition of Orphan Drug)
  - Subregulation 16I: Application for orphan drug designation
  - Subregulation 16J: Orphan Drug Designation
- Japan by:
  - Chapter 9-2, Article 77-2 of the Pharmaceutical Affairs Law

The orphan drug programs in the various countries are different in detail. They do have in common:

- Incentives and opportunities for the sponsor:
  - Fee reduction and / or tax reduction
  - Early building of close relationship with the agency
  - Market exclusivity for a certain period
- "The Price" to be paid by the Sponsor
  - Additional resources required in order to achieve the orphan drug status, e.g. provide documentation about the prevalence of the disease under discussion in the respective country
  - Annual reports to the authority
  - Financial disclosure to the authority obligatory
  - Orphan drug status can be lost if the financial benefit for the company is higher than expected
  - Market exclusivity can be lost if another product is clinically superior or the original orphan drug can not be supplied in sufficient quantity
  - Submission of a dossier for a "non-orphan drug" indication requires a different trade name

The Regulatory Affairs Manager has to evaluate the potential risks and benefits of the orphan drug status and include the final recommendation into his / her strategy.

4. REGULATORY STRATEGY

4.3 Definition of "Global Regulatory Strategy"

The definition provided in this section is not globally accepted or validated but only an individual attempt to define the concept of a regulatory strategy.

The regulatory strategy is one part of the Global Multidisciplinary Drug Development Strategy and supports the overall goals of the company in terms of successful submission / approval and ongoing successful maintenance of the marketed product. The information generated through regulatory intelligence serves as basis for the development of a regulatory strategy.

The regulatory strategy has to comply with the current regulatory legislation in the targeted regions. Therefore, it is advisable to develop a Global regulatory strategy and take that as a basis for the region or country specific strategy.

4.4 Regulatory Affairs Strategic Contributions to the Global Multidisciplinary Development Plan

This section describes the regulatory contributions to
- Competitor analysis and target labelling
- Definition of trade name and INN
- Definition of key markets
- Definition of a clinical development plan
- Identification and validation of relevant guidelines.

4.4.1 Competitor Analysis and Target Labelling

One major task of the global project team (with Regulatory Affairs as one discipline represented) is to evaluate competitors. This is a joint effort of Research, Marketing, Medicine, Regulatory Affairs departments and other disciplines if required. Research has a good impression of the research activities of other companies and universities (e.g. congresses, scientific publications, posters, press releases, share holder conferences, co-operations, personal network ...). Marketing identifies major competitors (companies, substance classes) that are already launched, their sales, their labelling etc. Regulatory Affairs provides regulatory data on the competitors The Medical Department finds out medically relevant details about the clinical development program of the competitors that have already been launched or are under development. For details see sections 3.1.2 and 3.1.3.

All these different pieces of information provided by different disciplines are brought together. They are the basis to define the target labelling of the product under development which has to be as competitive as possible. This includes e.g. formulation, dosages and regimen, application route, target population(s), indication, already known or suspected risks of this particular product or the substance class which might require additional investigations. The target labelling for the development candidate is updated as soon as new information becomes available (e.g. AEs from clinical studies, toxicological findings), and over the entire development period more disciplines get involved (e.g. drug safety for assessment of AEs and ADRs during the clinical development phases).

4.4.2 Definition of Trade Name and INN

Usually, definition of the trade name is a multidisciplinary attempt. Marketing does a market research to find the most beneficial trade name and trade dress. Regulatory Affairs makes sure that the trade name is in line with the corresponding guidelines for all the regions that plan to sell the future drug (based on the intelligence work). For details see section 3.1.2.

4.4.3 Definition of Key Markets

The Marketing Department provides information on the key markets which offer the best opportunities for a positive return on investment. The Medical Department assesses the particulars of the medical culture in the key countries that might have impact on the conduct of the clinical program (e.g. different competitors or different dosage regimens required in different countries). Regulatory Affairs provides knowledge about different regulatory requirements in different countries or regions in order to get the drug approved (based on the intelligence work).

The decision on the target regions and countries has to be taken as early as possible in order to adopt the development program accordingly. If a submission in Europe and Japan is planned the bridging concept (for details see section 3.3.1.1) needs to be planned as early as possible and agreed upon with the Japanese Health Authority. If submission in tropical regions is planned stability testing for climatic zones III and IV needs to be initiated as early as possible. These are only two examples to illustrate how the interdisciplinary driven decision where to launch has an immediate impact on the corresponding regulatory strategy.

4.4.4 Definition of a Clinical Development Plan

The Medical Department creates a clinical development plan which outlines all the studies that are assessed to be necessary until submission. The plan contains the clinical phase, study objectives, study designs, number of patients, participating countries, major investigators in the countries and timelines associated. Regulatory Affairs is requested to provide the Clinical Trial Applications for the planned studies in the respective countries, to provide the overview on guidelines for clinical development of the drug (e.g. guidelines for the development of an anti-asthma drug) and in addition to that indication-independent guidelines like the ones on QT-prolongation, ICH guideline on the conduct of a clinical trial / GCP etc. In addition, Regulatory Affairs provides an ongoing alerting service on current discussions within and between the agencies, upcoming guidelines, future developments of regulations. The contributions are based on the intelligence work described in the above sections.

4.4.5 Identification and Validation of Relevant Guidelines

In conjunction with the particulars of the product or the formulation (e.g. liposome formulation necessary for an intravenous drug), indication (e.g. asthma), target population(s) (e.g. children, elderly people), planned duration of the therapy (e.g. long term use) and the target regions / countries (e.g. USA, Europe and Australia), Regulatory Affairs provides the appropriate guidelines and makes sure that all disciplines involved do have the appropriate level of knowledge to work in accordance with regulatory requirements. In addition, Regulatory Affairs provides the "umbrella" of regulatory information (e.g. guidelines on how to conduct a clinical trial, guidelines on impurities) and proactively follows up with guidelines under development, current discussions, focus of interest of individual agencies etc.. It is part of the Regulatory Affairs strategy (and more concretely, regulatory intelligence) how to get the complete guideline picture.

Other facets of guideline identification and validation are:

- Is the product under development suitable for an orphan drug application
- Is the product under development suitable for a fast track condition
- Will there be an opportunity to get a waiver for the paediatric program (USA)
- Is there an opportunity to get a SPC in Europe after patent expiry
- ...

For details see section 3.3.3.

4.4.6 Life Cycle Management Strategy

Usually, after having successfully launched a product in the market, the company develops life cycle management strategies. Some examples for this are:

- Develop an i.v.-formulation after having developed an oral application. This is important e.g. for antibiotic drugs as those treatment regimes often foresee a sequential therapy: starting with an i.v.-application for some days during a life-threatening phase of the underlying infection and / intensive care unit treatment and then switch to oral treatment which can even be performed outside the hospital setting e.g. at home. This means developing the i.v.-formulation increases the number of indications covered.
- Develop a liquid formulation after having developed tablets. This development helps to include the paediatric and elderly populations that need mg/kg dosages and have difficulty swallowing solid dosage forms. The dosage required can be adopted to the individual and very different body weights of the paediatric patients.
- Develop an extended release tablet after the immediate release tablet. This is important e.g. for chronic diseases in older age classes as the change of the treatment regimen e.g. from tid to od increases patient compliance and helps to ensure the treatment success.

All these life cycle management activities need careful regulatory support. There are specific guidelines that need to be adhered to. Some modifications are completely new developments, others are variations, others are "extension applications" [23, 24]. The Regulatory Affairs Manager provides the knowledge about the necessary pre-requisites for these activities based on the intelligence work.

Other aspects of the product life cycle management are more "formally oriented" changes like relocation of production, change of excipients, increase the batch size, change of the production process etc. All of these processes need regulatory input regarding the authority requirements before implementing the changes.

4.5 Regulatory Strategy and Impact on other Disciplines

This section describes the regulatory strategies for

- Submission
- Health Authority Meetings
- Issue management.

4.5.1 Submission Strategy

Part of the regulatory strategy is the submission strategy. This covers for example the question if the centralised procedure or the mutual recognition procedure (MRP) is preferable in Europe. The final decision depends on the planned time of submission (the centralised procedure may become mandatory on a midterm basis for NMEs), the particulars of the product and the indication, the target countries for submission and the strength of the dossier (a weak dossier would always be a good reason for avoiding the centralised procedure). For products with a planned launch date after the enlargement of the European Union, it is also part of the strategic consideration how (if at all) to involve the Eastern European countries. This requires interaction with other disciplines like Marketing and Medical Department (different medical culture). For example, involvement of Eastern Europe needs marketing input as pricing will be affected and the re-import issue arises. Pre-requisite for these considerations is a carefully performed regulatory intelligence work so that information e.g. on the European enlargement and the current legal situation is available.

It is important to define the sequence of submissions in the various countries. It might for example be useful to submit first in the USA as many Asian and South American countries accept as the basis for their approval the US-NDA. Another reason may be that e.g. USA accepts 6 months stability data given the commitment that one year safety data is provided later, and Europe requires one year stability data at the time of submission. These aspects need to be agreed upon with the Medical Department (Medical needs to plan the studies accordingly) as well as with the Marketing Department (this discipline needs to plan the communication, publications etc. accordingly). A tabular overview structuring the timing of the planned submission should be created in accordance with the strategy chosen.

Planning of deficiency letter management also belongs to the submission strategy. Regulatory Affairs should be the single point of contact for the Health Authorities and receive the deficiency letter(s). Regulatory Affairs organises the answering process, defines timelines, checks consistency of the answers provided by the experts of the disciplines concerned, compiles the answers and communicates them to the authorities. As usually the time to answer the questions is limited the answering process should be pre-defined and availability of people within the key disciplines ensured during the critical period of time.

Another aspect of the regulatory submission strategy is the planning of the dossier composition. The CTD format is mandatory in the ICH regions since 1st of July 2003. Introduction into the local regulatory law is different; some countries granted transition periods to the applicants; some regions performed local adaptations (e.g. Japan). It has to be ensured that the regulatory requirements of the submitting countries are met. One also needs to consider the dossier preferences of Asian, South-American, Eastern European etc. countries as long as the CTD format is not yet globally mandatory.

A decision needs to be taken on electronic versus paper based submission. Even a CTD submission can be published both ways. If the decision is taken to publish electronically, eCTD versus CTD format needs to be decided. These decisions are usually taken together with the international project team (which includes the authoring disciplines) and the IT support function (publishing software available for electronic submission, authors and reviewers trained etc.). Hyperlinking / referencing has to be planned for paper based submissions as well as for electronic submissions (who, when, review, software support for hyperlinking). Regulatory has to have a plan in place how to assign the authors of the submission documents, how to ensure tracking of documents' completeness as well as adherence to the committed timelines, the review and quality control process of the submission and the final shipment of the dossier to the agencies.

All these submission related activities are performed in close co-operation with the global project team and mainly with the authoring disciplines like medicine, toxicology etc..

4.5.2 Strategy for Meetings with Health Authorities

According to the rules in the target regions / countries, Regulatory Affairs plans, organises and follows up with meetings with the corresponding Health Authorities (e.g. pre-IND meeting, end-of-phase-II-meeting, pre-launch meeting with the FDA, scientific advice from EMEA, advice from national Health Authorities). It is part of the regulatory strategy to define points in time when an authority contact is needed for a product under development. During drug development, there are two main types of authority meetings:

- Scientific advice meetings for clarification of specific issues (e.g. toxicology findings, choice of surrogate clinical endpoints, e.g. number of viruses for the development of an anti-viral compound, statistical analysis method) with the Health Authority
- "Formal Standard meetings" like pre-IND meetings, End-of-Phase I meetings, End-of-Phase II/III meetings and pre-NDA meetings / pre-submission meetings

The Health Authority meeting and general contact concepts differ between the regions. In Europe, Health Authority contact during the development phase of a product is limited, scientific advice is only provided if there is no guidance available for that type of question. The FDA maintains a constant contact with the sponsor over the entire drug development time and knows the product well when the NDA is submitted. Japan moves towards the FDA contact concept. These cultural differences need to be considered when planning multi-regional Health Authority meetings.

Timing of the scientific advice meetings is also critical. For example, one should seek scientific advice for a clinical development plan some time before performing the clinical phase of the drug development in order to make sure that the clinical development plan is accepted by the authority, that it is possible to implement the advice given into the clinical development plan and that the clinical studies under discussion in case of positive results will lead to a drug approval. It is part of the regulatory responsibility to alert the project team about the necessity of a scientific advice. For example, definition of the clinical endpoint is the main responsibility of the medical representative, but the Regulatory Affairs Manager has to know that this endpoint under discussion (e.g. number of viruses in the peripheral blood in the development of an anti-viral drug) is or is not covered by any guideline and needs agreement by the authority.

In Europe, several options for getting scientific advice are possible.
- Contact selected national Health Authorities in EU countries. The appropriate selection of these Health Authorities would be based on criteria like the Health Authority is a potential RMS / rapporteur for the development candidate, major experience in this indication available in that Health Authority, a very critical Health Authority that needs to be convinced about the quality of the development candidate as the Health Authority has major impact on pan-European decision making processes. Getting national advice is usually quicker than the EMEA scientific advice, but on the other hand national advice may vary between agencies and delay seeking central advice from the EMEA
- Request central scientific advice from the EMEA/CPMP. This approach ensures a consistent pan-European answer, but usually needs more time and is more cost-intensive than the national approach
- Seek national advice as a first step and after that seek EMEA advice in a second step

The FDA provides scientific advice according to the published rules (see below). Scientific advice meetings do not supersede the formal meetings mentioned above.

The consideration if the national advice is preferable over a CPMP advice in Europe is also part of the regulatory strategy. The final decision is usually taken in the project team and mainly with the disciplines involved in the specific interaction.

Depending on the subject (e.g. toxicological findings, clinical endpoints), Regulatory Affairs prepares the meeting and is supported by the specialists from the disciplines involved (e.g. toxicology, medicine); this includes the following aspects:
- Initial contact with the Health Authority presenting the request for a scientific advice with a presentation of the purpose of the meeting
- Meeting agenda
- Company participants (including external experts if applicable)
- Briefing documents (in accordance with the local Health Authority requirements)
- Organisation of the meeting (e.g. presentations, agenda, time needed for the meeting)

Regulatory Affairs organises the rehearsal ahead of the actual meeting, „orchestrates" the actual meeting with the authority and is responsible for the formal aspects (e.g. minutes). Even minor technical aspects like availability of a LCD projector and a computer for the presentations is essential for the successful rehearsal and Health Authority meeting and is the responsibility of the Regulatory Affairs Manager.

The following guidance documents are essential for planning and performing Health Authority meetings (the countries mentioned are examples for the variety of countries):

United States of America: Food and Drug Administration:

- Formal meetings with Sponsors and Applicants for PDUFA Products (February 2000)
- Formal Dispute Resolution: Appeals above the Division Level (February 2000)
- IND meetings for Human Drugs and Biologicals (Chemistry, Manufacturing and Controls): (February 2000)
- Advisory Committees: Implementing Section 120 of the Food and Drug Administration Modernization Act of 1997 (October 1998)
- Guidance on PMA Interactive Procedures for Day-100 meetings and Subsequent Deficiencies for Use By CDRH and Industry (February 19, 1998)
- Early Collaboration meetings Under the Food and Drug Administration Modernization Act: Guidance for Industry and CDRH Staff (February 19, 1998)

Europe (examples)

- EMEA Guidance for Companies Requesting Protocol Assistance regarding Scientific Advice (EMEA/H/238/02 Rev.1), June 2003
- Medicines and Healthcare Products Regulatory Agency: Provision of Pre-Application Scientific Advice for Human Medicinal Products by the Medicines and Healthcare products Regulatory Agency. 23 June 2003
- Wissenschaftliche und verfahrenstechnische Beratung durch das Bundes-Institut für Arzneimittel und Medizinprodukte (BfArM). Ergänzende Hinweise des BfArM zur Gemeinsamen Bekanntmachung des BfArM, BgVV und PEI vom 4.9.1998

4.5.3 Issue Management

During the drug development process, issues will happen from various perspectives. Some examples for issues are: the development candidate is not stable under the ICH-defined conditions, the tablet is too huge, the bitter taste can not be masked, critical toxicological findings, metabolism in humans is different from the animal models, the competitor drug has to be different in different regions, patient recruitment is difficult and slow.

All of the issues observed during the drug development need a thorough evaluation. Are there possible consequences from a regulatory perspective? An example for this would be: the company has seeked scientific advice from the EMEA in 2003, submission is planned for 2005, the EU-enlargement occurs in 2004. The issue would be that the accession countries have not been involved in the scientific advice procedure but will be part of the centralised European approval procedure. This increases the risk of an unsuccessful approval procedure. A mitigating action would be to carefully observe activities and opinions of the accession countries on an ongoing basis (part of the intelligence work) and alert the project team in case of significant events (e.g. negative vote on another development candidate of the same therapeutic area). A consequence might be to choose the MRP instead of the centralised procedure (if possible) or submit in early 2004 a subset of indications (if possible).

5. DISCUSSION

Traditionally, Regulatory Affairs has been perceived as a very cost-intensive "post office" that only takes the dossier and sends it to the Health Authority. This perception needs to be changed. Regulatory Affairs is one important discipline amongst others which supports the successful drug approval from very early development phases over the entire life-cycle of a product by providing regulatory knowledge to the global development team.

During the drug development phase, the regulatory strategy is one crucial success factor for the approval of the development candidate with the optimal labelling in the target countries. Submission and approval would not be possible without the appropriate dossier composition and without adherence to the respective guidance documents, the optimal labelling would not be feasible without scientific advice from Health Authorities that help us to design the optimal clinical development plan. These two examples already show some characteristics of the regulatory strategy: it is highly interactive with other disciplines (e.g. clinical development plan based on the scientific advice from a Health Authority which has been arranged according to the rules) and it is heavily based on thorough intelligence work (e.g. knowledge of relevant guidance documents) which enables the Regulatory Affairs Manager to handle the rules of the game and to develop the optimal regulatory strategy for the current development candidate. The pivotal basis for the regulatory strategy is the regulatory intelligence with all the facets mentioned in the previous sections of this document. Therefore, the time, workload and of course money invested in the regulatory intelligence work is well invested (on the expense side). Regulatory intelligence is one pre-requisite for the timely and successful drug approval, and that of course also translates back to money (on the income side). Therefore, regulatory intelligence may become a "sub-discipline" of the Regulatory Affairs discipline and develop a separate profile (e.g. more oriented towards Information Technology in terms of constantly handling information obtained via Internet).

Inadequate or missing intelligence information regarding the development candidate may lead to deficiency letters issued by the authorities as the documentation is incomplete or inadequate, and the company is under risk not getting approval for the drug or at least delaying the approval and launch of the product. This of course translates back to income lost, and usually the amount of these losses is higher than the investment into the appropriate intelligence work. Another example for the negative implications of inappropriate intelligence work would be the change of a production process that has been prepared (investing time and money) and then is refused by the authority due to non-adherence to the regulatory rules. An additional aspect is the perception of a company by the authority. Poorly compiled dossiers and inappropriately prepared scientific advice meetings will lead to an unfortunate perception of the company by the authority, which may have implications on future submissions.

The sources of regulatory intelligence knowledge do have different practical use for the Regulatory Affairs Manager. E.g. information or even guidance documents published by Health Authorities are of much greater importance and relevance than information published by trade associations or information provided during training sessions. When evaluating intelligence information, one should always rank the information according to the source, the level of importance, legal obligation and of course up to dateness.

6. REFERENCES

The Internet links provided in this document are meant as references for the respective sections and therefore not included into the list of references.

[1] GINA workshop report, Global Strategy for Asthma Management and Prevention, updated April 2002

[2] Wold Health Organization, Essential Drugs and Medicines Policy

[3] WHO Drug Information Vol 15, No. 2, 2001

[4] WHO Medicines Strategy: Framework for Action in Essential Drugs and medicines Policy 2002-2003 p. 45-46

[5] Council Regulations (EEC) No 2309/93 of 22 July 1993 laying down community procedures for the authorisation and supervision of medicinal products for human and veterinary use and establishing a European Agency for the Evaluation of Medicinal Products (Official Journal L 214, 24/08/1993 P. 0001 – 0021) as amended by Commission Regulation (EC) No. 649 / 98 of 23 March 1998 amending the annex to council regulation (EC) no. 649 / 98 of 23 March 1998 amending the annex to council regulation (EEC) No. 2309/93 (official journal L 088, 24/03/1998 P. 0007 – 0007)

[6] Pharmaceuticals in the European Union, European Commission 2000, http://pharmacos.eudra.org/F2/pharmacos/docs/brochure/pharmaeu.pdf

[7] EMEA (The European Agency for the Evaluation of Medicinal Products): Committee for proprietary medicinal products summary of opinion for KETEK – International Nonproprietary Name (INN) Telithromycin. CPMP/767/01: 29 March 2001

[8] EMEA (The European Agency for the Evaluation of Medicinal Products): Committee for proprietary medicinal products summary of opinion for LEVVIAX – International Nonproprietary Name (INN) Telithromycin. CPMP/972/01: 29 March 2001

[9] FDA (Food and Drug Administration): Advisory panel recommends FDA approval of KETEK® (telithromycin) tablets for treatment of community-acquired pneumonia – Innovative antibiotic is first in new class. Electronic version via Internet (Aventis Pharma AG): 2001

[10] DIRECTIVE 2001/83/EC OF THE EUROPEAN PARLIAMENT AND OF THE COUNCIL of 6 November 2001 on the Community code relating to medicinal products for human use

[11] DIRECTIVE 2001/20/EC OF THE EUROPEAN PARLIAMENT AND OF THE COUNCIL of 4 April 2001 on the approximation of the laws, regulations and administrative provisions of the Member States relating to the implementation of good clinical practice in the conduct of clinical trials on medicinal products for human use

[12] ICH Harmonised Tripartite Guideline: Organisation of the Common Technical Document for the Registration of Pharmaceuticals for Human Use (M4). Step 5 in September 2002. **EU** : Adopted by CPMP, November 2003, issued as CPMP/ICH/2887/99 rev.2 Organisation CTD. **MHLW**: : Adopted on July 1, 2003, PFSB/ELD Notification No. 0701004 (Revised Granularity to be notified)

[13] ICH eCTD Specification V 3.0 October 08 2002

[14] WHO/HTM/RBM/2003.50: assessment and monitoring of antimalarial drug efficacy for the treatment of uncomplicated falciparum malaria. WHO 2003

[15] International Conference on Harmonisation of technical requirements for registration of pharmaceuticals for human use: ICH Harmonised Guideline: Guideline for Good Clinical Practice E6. Recommended for adoption at step 4 of the ICH process on 1 May 1996 by the ICH steering committee

[16] International Conference on Harmonisation of technical requirements for registration of pharmaceuticals for human use: ICH Harmonised Guideline: Ethnic factors in the acceptability of foreign clinical data E5 Recommended for adoption at step 4 of the ICH process on 5 February 1998 by the ICH steering committee

[17]   ENGLISH REGULATORY INFORMATION TASK FORCE, JPMA. Pharmaceutical Administration and Regulations in Japan (March 2003)

[18]   CPMP/EWP/558/95 rev 1: Note for guidance on evaluation of medicinal products indicated for treatment of bacterial infections. Draft. Deadline for comments November 2003

[19]   CPMP/EWP/2655/99: Points to consider on pharmacokinetics and pharmacodynamics in the development of antibacterial medicinal products, 2000

[20]   Concept paper on the development of the revision of the committee for the proprietary medicinal products (CPMP) note for guidance (NFG) on evaluation of new anti-bacterial medicinal products (CPMP/EWP/588/95) and the CPMP NFG on the pharmacodynamic sections of the SPC for anti-bacterial medicinal products (CPMP/EWP/520/96). [CPMP/EWP/1412/01]

[21]   Guidance for Industry: Developing antimicrobial drugs – general considerations for clinical trials. Draft Guidance, July 1998

[22]   Guidance for Industry – Points to consider. Division of Anti-Infective Drug Products, 1997

[23]   COMMISSION REGULATION (EC) No 1084/2003 of 3 June 2003 concerning the examination of variations to the terms of a marketing authorisation for medicinal products for human use and veterinary medicinal products granted by a competent authority of a Member State] AND [14]

[24]   COMMISSION REGULATION (EC) No 1085/2003 of 3 June 2003 concerning the examination of variations to the terms of a marketing authorisation for medicinal products for human use and veterinary medicinal products falling within the scope of Council Regulation (EEC) No 2309/93